Breaking Free from Sugar: A Complete Guide to Reducing Sugar for a Healthier Life

Cut Sugar, Curb Cravings, and Rediscover Your Natural Energy
Sugar Detox

Evelyn R. Beacham

"Breaking Free from Sugar: A Complete Guide to Reducing Sugar for a Healthier Life" is your essential roadmap to transforming your relationship with sugar. Designed for those ready to cut sugar and curb cravings, this comprehensive guide provides practical strategies to help you reduce sugar in your diet, break free from sugar addiction, and restore your natural energy. Discover easy-to-follow steps for a sugar detox, tips on managing cravings, and insights into how sugar impacts both body and mind. Packed with expert advice, science-backed methods, and lifestyle tips, this book empowers you to take control of your health and live a life less dependent on sugar. Whether you're looking to lose weight, boost your energy, or improve overall wellness, *Breaking Free from Sugar* offers the tools and encouragement to succeed. Start your journey to a healthier, balanced, and more vibrant you!

CONTENTS

You will find help within this book to cope
with:

- Sugar detox
- Reducing sugar intake
- Beating sugar cravings
- Sugar addiction recovery
- Healthy diet transformation
- Natural energy boost
- Sugar-free lifestyle

Why Sugar is the 'Sweet Enemy'

The Addictive Nature of Sugar: A Hidden Obsession

I didn't always realize just how addictive sugar could be. At first, it felt innocent—just a cookie here, a sweetened latte there. But over time, I noticed something unsettling: the more sugar I had, the more I *wanted*. And if I didn't get it, I'd feel moody, restless, and tired. What I didn't know back then was that sugar works a lot like a drug—it taps into the same reward system in your brain, releasing dopamine and making you feel good.

But there's a catch. Just like with other addictions, your brain builds up a tolerance, so you need more sugar to feel the same sense of satisfaction. Before I knew it, I was on a rollercoaster of sugar highs and crashes—one minute buzzing with energy, the next slumped on the couch, reaching for something sugary to perk me up again. I was stuck in a vicious cycle, and I didn't even realize how much control sugar had over me.

I also discovered that sugar is hidden in everything. It's not just in candy or desserts; it sneaks into foods we think are healthy—things like granola, yogurt, smoothies, even bread. It's disguised under dozens of names like dextrose, maltodextrin, agave, or corn syrup. The food industry loves sugar because it's addictive, and it keeps us coming back for more.

My Personal Story: Breaking Free from Sugar's Grip

For years, sugar was my go-to comfort. If I was tired, stressed, or bored, I'd grab something sweet. A chocolate bar mid-afternoon. A muffin with my morning coffee. Ice cream at the end of a long day. I told myself it was no big deal—*"Everyone has a sweet tooth, right?"* But deep down, I knew something wasn't right. I started to notice that I wasn't just enjoying these treats—I was depending on them.

I tried to quit a few times. I'd wake up determined, only to find myself sneaking a cookie by noon, telling myself, *"Just one won't hurt."* That "one" cookie would quickly turn into a binge. The cravings were so powerful that it felt impossible to say no. Then, one night, I sat on my couch with a pint of ice cream and, before I even knew it, I'd eaten the entire thing. I wasn't even hungry—I was just numb. And instead of feeling satisfied, I felt guilty and trapped. That was the moment I knew something had to change.

I wasn't just addicted to sugar—I was stuck in a toxic relationship with it. It gave me temporary joy but left me feeling drained, dependent, and out of control. That's when I made a promise to myself: I was going to break up with sugar for good.

My Mission: Breaking Free and Reclaiming My Health

This book is the result of my journey—and I want it to be your guide as well. I've been where you are, and I know how hard it can feel to walk away from something that's been a constant in your life. But I also know this: you don't have to be a slave to sugar anymore. You can take back control, and I'm going to show you how.

This journey isn't just about quitting sugar—it's about reclaiming your health, your energy, and your sense of well-being. Once you get off the sugar rollercoaster, life feels so much better. You sleep better. Your mood stabilizes. Your cravings fade away. And perhaps best of all, you start to feel in control of your body and your choices.

I know it sounds hard, but here's the good news: You don't have to do it perfectly, and you don't have to do it alone. This isn't about deprivation—it's about freedom. It's about freeing yourself from the highs and lows that come with sugar and discovering a way to feel good without needing a quick fix.

What You Can Expect from This Book

This book isn't just another diet plan. It's a step-by-step guide to breaking free from sugar's grip and creating a life that feels sweet without needing a constant sugar hit. Here's what you'll find inside:

1. **Education and Awareness:**
    I'll walk you through how sugar affects your body and mind, why it can feel so addictive, and how to spot hidden sugars in the foods you eat every day.

2. **Practical Strategies:**
    Together, we'll create a detox plan that works for you—whether you want to quit sugar all at once or take it step-by-step. I'll show you how to manage cravings, avoid relapses, and stay motivated, even on tough days.

3. **Delicious Recipes and Meal Plans:**
    I get it—food should be enjoyable. So I've included simple, delicious recipes that are

free from added sugars but still satisfying. You'll find everything from breakfasts and snacks to sugar-free desserts that you'll actually look forward to eating.

4. **Mindset Shifts:**
   Breaking up with sugar isn't just about what's on your plate—it's about changing your relationship with food. We'll dive into the emotional side of eating and explore mindful practices that help you stay connected to your body and its real needs.

5. **Encouragement and Accountability:**
   I've included journaling exercises, habit trackers, and real-life success stories to keep you motivated. Plus, you'll find tips on how to handle social situations and celebrations without feeling deprived.

A Sneak Peek at What's Ahead

I know the idea of giving up sugar might feel overwhelming, but don't worry—we're going to take it one step at a time. In the next chapter, we'll dive into the hidden sugars lurking in your kitchen and learn how to spot them, even when they're disguised as "healthy" ingredients. You'll be surprised how many foods you thought were harmless are actually loaded with added sugars!

You Can Do This—And I'll Be With You Every Step of the Way

I'm not here to tell you this will be easy. Quitting sugar takes effort and commitment. There will be moments when you'll want to give in—and that's okay. This journey isn't about perfection; it's about progress.

But I can promise you this: It's worth it On the other side of those cravings and crashes is a life that feels lighter, more balanced, and genuinely sweet. And you're not doing this alone—I'll be with you, guiding you every step of the way.

This is your chance to reclaim your energy, your health, and your happiness. You deserve to feel good. And together, we're going to make that happen.

Understanding the Science of Sugar

How Sugar Affects the Brain: Dopamine Release and Addiction

When we eat sugar, something powerful happens inside our brains—**dopamine**, the neurotransmitter responsible for feelings of pleasure and reward, is released. It's the same chemical that lights up when we experience joy or accomplish something exciting, like winning a game or getting a compliment. This instant "feel-good" hit from sugar makes us feel temporarily satisfied, happy, or comforted. But here's the problem:

- **The more sugar you consume, the more your brain adapts**, reducing the amount of dopamine it releases over time. This leads to **tolerance**, which means you need more and more sugar to feel the same sense of pleasure.

- Over time, **sugar hijacks your reward system**, much like addictive substances do. The more frequently you indulge, the more dependent you become on sugary foods to feel okay. This is why cravings can feel so overwhelming—it's not just in your head; your brain is actively seeking its next fix.

- Sugar also **disrupts the balance of neurotransmitters** involved in mood regulation. A sugary binge might make you feel euphoric for a moment, but once your dopamine levels crash, you're left feeling irritable, anxious, or even depressed—fueling the cycle of craving more sugar to escape those lows.

Types of Sugar: Natural vs. Added Sugars

Not all sugars are created equal. There's a big difference between **naturally occurring sugars** found in whole foods and the **added sugars** found in processed products. Here's how they stack up:

1. **Natural Sugars**:

o **Fructose**: Found in fruits. When consumed in whole fruits, fructose is accompanied by **fiber, vitamins, and antioxidants**, which slow down the absorption of sugar and help your body process it more efficiently.

o **Lactose**: Found in dairy products like milk and yogurt. It's broken down slowly in the body and provides a more stable source of energy.

o **Natural sugars are less likely to cause spikes and crashes** because the fiber or protein in these foods keeps blood sugar levels stable.

2. **Added Sugars**:

o **Sucrose (table sugar)**: A combination of glucose and fructose. It's highly processed and rapidly absorbed by the body, causing a **quick spike in blood sugar** followed by a crash.

o **High-Fructose Corn Syrup (HFCS)**: Found in sodas, candies, and processed foods. HFCS is cheaper than sugar and even more addictive. It **bypasses the liver's regulation process**, leading to excess fat storage and metabolic issues.

o **Agave Syrup, Maltodextrin, and More**: Often marketed as healthy alternatives, but these sugars behave much like regular table sugar when it comes to spiking blood sugar levels.

Understanding these differences helps you make **informed choices** about where your sugar is coming from. While natural sugars in

whole foods aren't harmful in moderation, **added sugars**—especially in processed foods—are the real culprits behind many health problems.

Hidden Sugars in Common Foods and Misleading Labels

Even if you think you're avoiding sugar, it's probably sneaking into your diet. **Food manufacturers often hide sugar under different names** to make products seem healthier than they are. Here's what you need to know:

- **Sugar by Another Name**: Look out for these common aliases: maltodextrin, dextrose, cane syrup, fructose, agave nectar, glucose, and barley malt.

  "Healthy" Foods Loaded with Sugar: Foods like flavored yogurt, granola bars, protein shakes, salad dressings, and even whole-grain breads often contain added sugars. A **single serving** of flavored yogurt can contain as much sugar as a candy bar!

- **Misleading Labels**:

    o Products labeled as "low-fat" or "diet" often **compensate for the lack of fat with extra sugar** to maintain taste.

    o Even foods labeled "organic" or "natural" can contain large amounts of sugar.

    o Be wary of serving sizes: Many products use **small serving sizes** to make it look like they contain less sugar than they actually do. For example, a cereal box might list 5 grams of sugar per serving, but the serving size is only half a cup—far less than most people eat.

Learning to **read food labels carefully** is key to avoiding hidden sugars. Look for ingredients ending in "-ose" and watch out for **products with more than one type of added sugar**.

The Connection Between Sugar and Chronic Diseases

Sugar doesn't just affect your weight—it can have serious long-term effects on your health. When consumed in excess, sugar is linked to several chronic diseases, including:

1. **Diabetes**:

    o Consistently high sugar intake leads to **insulin resistance**, where your cells stop responding to insulin, making it harder for your body to manage blood sugar levels. This increases your risk of **Type 2 diabetes**.

2. **Heart Disease**:

    o Sugar contributes to **chronic inflammation**, which is a major risk factor for heart disease. Excess sugar also raises **triglyceride levels** and promotes the buildup of **fat around your organs** (visceral fat), both of which increase your risk of heart attacks.

3. **Obesity**:

    o Excess sugar gets stored as **fat in the liver** and around the abdomen, leading to weight gain and obesity. Sugary foods and drinks **disrupt hunger hormones**, making you feel hungry sooner and causing you to overeat.

4. **Non-Alcoholic Fatty Liver Disease (NAFLD)**:

    o High intake of fructose and other

sugars **overloads the liver**, leading to fat buildup, which can progress to liver disease.

Reducing sugar isn't just about **losing weight**—it's about **protecting your long-term health** and lowering your risk of these life-threatening conditions.

How Sugar Impacts Mental Health: Anxiety, Depression, and Mood Swings

Sugar doesn't just take a toll on your body—it also affects your **mental well-being**.

1. **Mood Swings and Emotional Instability**:

    o   Sugar causes **sharp spikes in blood glucose**, followed by rapid crashes. These fluctuations can lead to **irritability, anxiety, and brain fog**. It's common to feel euphoric after a sugar binge, only to crash into a low mood a short time later.

    o   This pattern can leave you feeling **out of control emotionally**, making it harder to manage stress or stay focused throughout the day.

2. **The Link Between Sugar and Depression**:

   o Several studies have found a **strong correlation between sugar consumption and depression**. Excess sugar **increases inflammation** in the brain, which has been linked to depressive symptoms.

   o Over time, the body's constant blood sugar swings and insulin resistance may also **disrupt serotonin production**, affecting mood regulation and increasing the risk of anxiety and depression.

3. **Increased Risk of Anxiety**:

   o Sugar stimulates the release of cortisol, the stress hormone. This can make **existing anxiety worse** and trigger feelings of restlessness or panic. If you're prone to anxiety, sugary foods can leave you feeling worse, not better.

4. **Brain Fog and Poor Focus**:

o When your blood sugar drops after a spike, it becomes harder to concentrate or stay productive. Many people describe this as **"brain fog"**—a state of sluggish thinking where even simple tasks feel overwhelming.

Learning to reduce sugar intake can lead to **better emotional stability, clearer thinking, and more balanced energy** throughout the day.

How to Wean Off Sugar Gradually

Cold Turkey vs. Gradual Detox: Which One is Right for You?

When it comes to quitting sugar, there are **two main approaches**—going cold turkey or following a gradual detox. Both have their pros and cons, and the key is finding the method that works best for your lifestyle and personality.

- **Cold Turkey Detox:**

o   **What It Is**: You quit sugar all at once—no exceptions, no cheat days.

o   **Pros**: Faster results; removes temptation entirely, reducing cravings over time.

o   **Cons**: Can trigger intense withdrawal symptoms (headaches, fatigue, irritability); harder to stick with if you rely on sugar for emotional comfort.

o   **Best For**: People who thrive on structure, are highly motivated, or want to make a dramatic lifestyle change.

- **Gradual Detox**:

o   **What It Is**: You reduce sugar intake slowly by cutting back on certain foods over time.

o   **Pros**: Easier to maintain long-term; fewer withdrawal symptoms; allows time to build new habits gradually.

o   **Cons**: Results take longer, and it may feel like progress is slow.

o   **Best For**: People who prefer slow, sustainable changes or those who struggle with intense cravings.

Tip: If you're not sure which approach suits you, try combining the two—**start with a gradual reduction** for a week or two, then switch to a more structured cold-turkey approach when you feel ready.

The First 7 Days: Overcoming Withdrawal Symptoms

The first week of detoxing is often the most difficult. As your body adjusts to life without sugar, **withdrawal symptoms** can set in, but don't worry—these are temporary! Knowing what to expect and having strategies to manage these symptoms will make all the difference.

- **Day 1–3: The Adjustment Period**

    o **What You May Feel**: Headaches, irritability, sugar cravings, and brain fog. You might also experience fatigue as your body adjusts to the absence of quick sugar energy.

    o **What's Happening**: Your blood sugar levels are stabilizing, and your brain is adjusting to the lack of dopamine spikes from sugar.

    o **How to Cope**:

        ▪ Drink plenty of water to stay hydrated and reduce

headaches.

- Eat meals rich in **fiber, protein, and healthy fats** to keep blood sugar levels stable.

- Consider herbal teas or sparkling water as replacements for sugary

drinks.

- **Day 4–7: Breaking Through the Fog**

  o **What You May Feel**: Cravings might intensify during this period, and you may feel a bit sluggish. Some people report minor mood swings or trouble sleeping.

  o **What's Happening**: Your insulin levels are stabilizing, and your liver is working to regulate glycogen stores. The cravings mean your brain is still adjusting to life without sugar's quick rewards.

  o **How to Cope**:

    - Keep **healthy snacks** like nuts, seeds, and fruit handy to combat cravings.

- Use distractions—exercise, go for a walk, or engage in a hobby when cravings strike.

- Practice **mindful eating**: Pause before giving in to cravings and ask yourself if you're really hungry, thirsty or just bored.

Key Tip: Be gentle with yourself. Withdrawal symptoms are **normal** and won't last forever. By Day 7, most people begin to feel more energized and stable.

Setting SMART Goals for a Sugar Detox

One of the most effective ways to stay on track is by setting **SMART goals**—Specific, Measurable, Achievable, Relevant, and Time-bound. Here are some examples tailored for a sugar detox:

- **Specific**: "I will stop adding sugar to my morning coffee starting tomorrow."

- **Measurable**: "I'll track my sugar intake and reduce it to 25 grams or less per day within two weeks."

- **Achievable**: "I'll switch to natural sweeteners like stevia or monk fruit instead of sugar for the next 30 days."

- **Relevant**: "Reducing sugar will help me feel more energetic and focused throughout the day."

- **Time-bound**: "I'll commit to following a sugar-free diet for the next 30 days."

Tip: Write your goals down in a **journal or planner** to hold yourself accountable. Regularly review and adjust them if necessary—progress isn't always linear, and that's okay.

Tracking Progress: Journals, Apps, or Daily Reflections

Tracking your progress not only keeps you accountable but also helps you **notice patterns** and stay motivated. There are a few ways to do this:

1. **Journaling**:

   o Write a short daily entry tracking how you feel emotionally and physically.

   o Log cravings, energy levels, and any

slip-ups (without guilt—just observe them).

- o Reflect on how your body and mood change throughout the detox process.

2. **Apps and Tools:**

- o Use apps like **MyFitnessPal, Yazio, or Sugar Tracker** to monitor your sugar intake and track your meals.

- o Habit-tracking apps like **Habitica or Streaks** can help you build momentum with daily goals.

- o Some apps provide **notifications and reminders** to drink water or log your meals, making it easier to stay on track.

3. **Daily Reflections:**

- o Take a few minutes every night to **rate your day**—How did you feel? What challenges did you face? What went well?

- o Use these reflections to **identify triggers** that make you crave sugar (stress, boredom, social events) and brainstorm healthier coping mechanisms.

A Timeline: What Happens to Your Body Without Sugar?

This timeline will help you stay motivated by showing what to expect as your body adjusts to life without sugar.

- **After 1 Week**:

    o Your **blood sugar levels stabilize**, and cravings begin to decrease.

    o You may notice an improvement in **energy levels**—no more afternoon crashes.

    o Mood swings become less intense as your brain adjusts to steady energy levels.

    o If you've struggled with bloating or water retention, you may feel lighter.

- **After 2 Weeks**:

    o Cravings become **less frequent** and

easier to manage.

o Your taste buds may **reset**, making naturally sweet foods like fruits taste more flavorful.

o You'll likely experience **improved digestion**, with less bloating or discomfort.

o Many people report **better sleep** and clearer thinking, as sugar-related brain fog lifts.

- **After 1 Month**:

o You'll feel **more in control** of your food choices, with fewer emotional triggers for sugar.

o Your **skin may improve**, as reduced sugar intake can lead to fewer breakouts and less inflammation.

o You may have lost a few pounds if weight loss was part of your goal, thanks to reduced sugar-induced snacking and cravings.

o Mentally, you'll feel **more stable and positive**, with fewer mood swings or anxious moments.

Long-Term Benefits: If you maintain your sugar detox beyond the first month, you'll reduce your risk of chronic illnesses like diabetes, heart disease, and obesity. Your body will continue to operate more efficiently, with **balanced hormones, steady energy, and improved mental clarity**.

Key Takeaways for a Successful Sugar Detox

- **Plan ahead**: Know what meals and snacks you'll rely on to avoid reaching for sugar.

- **Stay hydrated**: Thirst is often mistaken for hunger or cravings.

- **Don't aim for perfection**: Slip-ups happen—what matters is getting back on track.
- **Celebrate small wins**: Every day without sugar is a step toward better health—acknowledge your progress!

Identifying Emotional Eating Patterns

Emotional eating occurs when individuals use food to cope with feelings instead of hunger. Here are ways to recognize these patterns:

- **Keep a Food Journal:** Track what you eat, when you eat, and your feelings during meals or snacks. Note emotional triggers (e.g., stress, boredom) and any patterns that arise over time. This can reveal associations between emotions and eating habits.

- **Self-Reflection Questions:**

    o What emotions do I experience before I eat?

o Am I eating out of hunger or as a response to an emotional trigger?

o How do I feel after I eat? Am I satisfied or guilty?

- **Body Awareness:** Pay attention to physical sensations in your body. Are you feeling tense, anxious, or fatigued? Recognizing these signs can help distinguish between emotional hunger and physical hunger.

3. How Stress, Boredom, and Emotional Triggers Fuel Sugar Cravings

Understanding the psychological factors behind cravings can empower individuals to address them:

- **Stress:** High-stress levels lead to increased cortisol production, which can enhance cravings for sugary and fatty foods. These foods may provide temporary relief and comfort but can lead to a cycle of dependency and guilt.

- **Boredom:** Eating can serve as a distraction from boredom. Individuals may reach for snacks out of habit rather than hunger. This is often associated with mindless eating while watching TV or scrolling through devices.

- **Emotional Triggers:** Feelings such as sadness, loneliness, or anxiety often lead to cravings for comfort foods, which are typically high in sugar. This creates a cycle where individuals seek food to soothe emotional pain, leading to guilt or shame later.

4. Mindful Eating Practices to Break the Habit

Mindful eating focuses on being present during meals, enhancing awareness of food choices and the eating experience:

- **Eat Slowly and Savor:** Take time to chew and enjoy each bite. This can enhance satisfaction and help individuals recognize when they are full.

- **Eliminate Distractions:** Avoid eating in front of screens. Create a dedicated eating environment to foster mindfulness.

- **Focus on Sensations:** Pay attention to flavors, textures, and aromas. This practice can deepen your relationship with food and reduce emotional eating.

- **Check In with Yourself:** Before reaching for a snack, pause and ask yourself: Am I hungry? What am I feeling right now? This moment of reflection can prevent mindless eating.

5. Alternatives to Emotional Snacking

Finding alternatives to cope with emotions can reduce reliance on food:

- **Journaling:** Write about feelings, thoughts, and experiences. This can help process emotions without turning to food. Consider prompts like:
    - o What am I feeling right now?
    - o What triggered this emotion?
    - o How can I address this feeling constructively?

- **Exercise:** Physical activity is a powerful mood booster. It releases endorphins, which can alleviate stress and improve overall well-being. Find activities you enjoy, whether it's walking, yoga, dancing, or a workout class.

- **Breathing Exercises:** Deep breathing can reduce stress and anxiety. Try techniques like the 4-7-8 breathing method:

    0. **Inhale deeply through your nose for 4 counts.**

    1. **Hold your breath for 7 counts.**

    2. **Exhale slowly through your mouth for 8 counts.**

Practicing this for a few minutes can help

refocus your mind and calm your body.

5. Behavioral Techniques: Habit Replacement and Reward Systems
Creating healthier habits involves replacing unhealthy behaviors with positive alternatives:

- **Habit Replacement:**

    o Identify specific situations where you typically eat emotionally (e.g., watching TV, feeling stressed).

    o Replace the eating behavior with a healthier action. For instance, when you feel the urge to snack, consider drinking a glass of water, taking a walk, or doing a quick stretch.

- **Reward Systems:** Establish a reward system for yourself to reinforce positive behaviors:

    o **Set small, achievable goals (e.g., a week of mindful eating).**

    o **Reward yourself with non-food treats, such as a movie night, a new book, or a spa day, rather than food-based rewards.**

Additional Strategies and Ideas

- **Support Systems:** Engage with friends, family, or support groups who understand your journey. Sharing experiences can provide motivation and accountability.

- **Educational Resources:** Consider reading books or taking courses on emotional eating and mindful practices to deepen your understanding and strategies.

- **Professional Help:** If emotional eating becomes overwhelming, consider seeking help from a therapist or nutritionist specializing in emotional eating.

- **Practice Self-Compassion:** Recognize that everyone experiences emotional eating at times. Rather than berating yourself, practice self-compassion and understanding. This mindset can help reduce guilt and promote healthier choices.

By combining these strategies, you can cultivate a healthier relationship with food, improve emotional well-being, and reduce

reliance on food for comfort. Each step taken towards understanding and managing emotional eating contributes to a more balanced and fulfilling life.

34

Reshaping Your Relationship with Food

Creating a healthier and more fulfilling relationship with food involves understanding your body's needs, redefining indulgence, and cultivating new habits. Here's a deeper exploration of various aspects to consider:

1. Enjoying Sweetness Without Sugar
Fruits: Nature's Candy

- **Fresh Fruits:** Incorporate a variety of fruits like berries, apples, and citrus, which are naturally sweet and rich in vitamins, fiber, and antioxidants. They can satisfy sweet cravings and provide essential nutrients.

- **Dried Fruits:** Options like apricots, figs, and dates offer concentrated sweetness, but be mindful of portion sizes as they are calorie-dense.

- **Frozen Fruits:** Perfect for smoothies or as a frozen treat. Consider blending bananas with a splash of almond milk for a creamy, ice-cream-like texture.

Spices and Flavor Enhancers

- **Cinnamon:** This spice not only adds warmth and sweetness without sugar but also helps regulate blood sugar levels. Sprinkle it on oatmeal, yogurt, or roasted vegetables.

- **Vanilla Extract:** Adds a sweet aroma and flavor to dishes. Use it in smoothies, baked goods, or oatmeal.
- Nutmeg and Ginger: These spices can enhance sweet flavors without adding sugar, perfect for pumpkin dishes or smoothies.

Healthier Alternatives

- **Natural Sweeteners:** Consider using honey, maple syrup, or agave in moderation. Stevia and monk fruit extract are zero-calorie alternatives that can sweeten without the negative impacts of refined sugar.

- **Greek Yogurt with Honey:** Mix Greek yogurt with a drizzle of honey and a sprinkle of nuts for a nutritious dessert that feels indulgent.

- **Nut Butters**: Almond or peanut butter can add richness and a hint of sweetness to snacks like apple slices or rice cakes.

3. Understanding Hunger vs. Craving

Listening to Your Body's Signals

- **Mindful Eating:** Pay attention to physical hunger cues (e.g., stomach growling, energy levels) versus emotional cues (e.g., stress, boredom). Take time to assess how you feel before reaching for food.

- **Food Journaling:** Keep a journal to track what you eat, how you feel, and your hunger levels. This practice can help you identify patterns and triggers for cravings.

- **Wait 20 Minutes:** When you think you're hungry, wait for 20 minutes to see if the feeling persists. This can help distinguish true hunger from cravings driven by emotions or boredom.

Strategies to Differentiate

- **Hydration Check:** Sometimes thirst can masquerade as hunger. Drink a glass of water before reaching for a snack.

- **Healthy Snacking:** If you're not truly hungry but still crave something, opt for healthier snacks like carrot sticks, nuts, or air-popped popcorn.

3. Rethinking "Treats" and Indulgences
Shift in Mindset

- **Reframe Treats:** Instead of viewing treats as rewards for good behavior, see them as part of a balanced lifestyle. Consider treats that nourish rather than just indulge.

- **Savoring:** Practice mindful eating by taking small bites of a treat and savoring each one. This can lead to greater satisfaction and a reduced desire to overindulge.

Healthy Indulgences

- **Homemade Alternatives:** Experiment with recipes that use natural sweeteners and whole ingredients. For example, make banana oat cookies or chia seed pudding.

- **Portion Control:** Allow yourself to enjoy treats, but keep portions small. Instead of a large piece of cake, opt for a mini version or a few bites to satisfy your sweet tooth.

4. **Rewiring Habits:** Forming New Rituals Around Meals and Snacks

Creating New Rituals

- **Meal Preparation:** Dedicate time each week to prepare meals and snacks. This can help you make healthier choices and reduce impulsive eating.

- **Mindful Meal Times:** Set aside time for meals without distractions (like TV or smartphones). Focus on the taste, texture, and aroma of your food.

Building Healthy Habits

- **Snacking Rituals**: Instead of reaching for chips or sweets, create a habit of preparing healthy snacks ahead of time. Try hummus with veggies or whole grain crackers with guacamole.

- **Celebrate Nourishment:** Shift focus from food as a reward to food as nourishment. Incorporate rituals like expressing gratitude before meals or sharing food with family and friends to enhance your eating experience.

Incorporating Movement

- **Active Meals:** Combine meals with physical activity. Consider taking a walk after dinner or engaging in fun, active family outings that encourage a healthy lifestyle.

Conclusion

Reshaping your relationship with food is an ongoing journey. By understanding and embracing natural sweetness, listening to your body's cues, redefining indulgences, and establishing new habits, you can cultivate a healthier, more satisfying approach to eating. This transformation not only enhances your physical health but also promotes a positive mental outlook on food.

6 MEAL PLANS

Here's a comprehensive 7-day meal plan designed for beginners who want to follow a sugar-free lifestyle. This plan focuses on simple, easy-to-follow recipes for breakfasts, snacks, desserts, and tips for cooking with low-glycemic index foods. Each day includes meal ideas that minimize added sugars while maximizing flavor and nutrition.

7-Day Sugar-Free Meal Plan

Day 1

Breakfast:
- **Avocado Toast with Eggs**
    - o Whole-grain or sprouted bread topped with smashed avocado, poached eggs, salt, pepper, and a sprinkle of chili flakes.

Snack:
- **Roasted Almonds**
    - o Toss raw almonds with olive oil, sea salt, and your favorite spices. Roast at 350°F (175°C) for 10–15 minutes.

Lunch:
- **Quinoa Salad**
    - o Cooked quinoa mixed with diced cucumbers, cherry tomatoes, red onion, parsley, olive oil, lemon juice, salt, and pepper.

Snack:
- **Veggie Chips**
    - o Thinly slice vegetables like sweet potatoes, beets, or zucchini, toss with olive oil, salt, and bake until crispy.

Dinner:
- **Baked Lemon Herb Chicken**
    - o Chicken breasts marinated in lemon juice, garlic, and herbs, then baked. Serve with steamed broccoli and brown rice.

Day 2

Breakfast:
- **Chia Seed Pudding**
  - Mix 1/4 cup chia seeds with 1 cup unsweetened almond milk and a splash of vanilla extract. Let it sit overnight. Top with fresh berries in the morning.

Snack:
- **Apple Slices with Almond Butter**
  - Sliced apples served with a side of natural almond butter.

Lunch:
- **Lentil Soup**
  - Cook lentils with carrots, celery, onions, and vegetable broth. Season with herbs like thyme and bay leaf.

Snack:
- **Cucumber Slices with Hummus**
  - Fresh cucumber slices dipped in homemade or store-bought hummus.

Dinner:
- **Stuffed Bell Peppers**
  - Bell peppers stuffed with a mixture of ground turkey, black beans, corn, diced tomatoes, and spices. Bake until the peppers are tender.

Day 3
Breakfast:
- **Smoothie Bowl**
  - Blend spinach, banana, and unsweetened almond milk. Pour into a bowl and top with sliced fruit,

nuts, and seeds.

Snack:
- **Energy Balls**
    - o Mix rolled oats, nut butter, flax seeds, and chopped dates. Roll into balls and refrigerate.

Lunch:
- **Greek Salad**
    - o Chopped cucumbers, tomatoes, red onion, olives, and feta cheese, dressed with olive oil and oregano.

Snack:
- **Roasted Chickpeas**
    - o Toss canned chickpeas with olive oil, salt, and spices. Roast until crunchy.

Dinner:
- **Zucchini Noodles with Pesto**
    - o Spiralize zucchini and toss with homemade basil pesto and grilled chicken.

Day 4
Breakfast:
- **Egg Muffins**
    - o Whisk eggs with diced vegetables (spinach, bell peppers, onions) and bake in muffin tins.

Snack:
- **Celery Sticks with Cream Cheese**
    - o Celery sticks filled with cream cheese or nut butter.

Lunch:
- **Tuna Salad Lettuce Wraps**
    - o Tuna mixed with avocado and Greek

yogurt, served in large lettuce leaves.

Snack:

- **Hard-Boiled Eggs**
    - o Simple, protein-packed snack seasoned with salt and pepper.

Dinner:

- **Cauliflower Rice Stir-Fry**
    - o Cauliflower rice stir-fried with mixed vegetables, tofu or chicken, and soy sauce or tamari.

Day 5
Breakfast:

- **Overnight Oats**
    - o Combine rolled oats, unsweetened almond milk, chia seeds, and a pinch of cinnamon. Let sit overnight and top with nuts in the morning.

Snack:

- **Nut Mix**
    - o A mix of unsalted walnuts, pecans, and pumpkin seeds.

Lunch:

- **Grilled Vegetable Salad**
    - o Grilled zucchini, bell peppers, and asparagus on a bed of greens with a balsamic vinaigrette.

Snack:

- **Bell Pepper Strips**
    - o Fresh bell pepper strips served with guacamole.

Dinner:

- **Baked Salmon with Asparagus**

o Salmon fillet seasoned with lemon, garlic, and herbs, baked alongside asparagus.

Day 6
Breakfast:
- **Smoothie**
    - o Blend spinach, coconut milk, frozen berries, and a scoop of protein powder.

Snack:
- **Kale Chips**
    - o Toss kale with olive oil and sea salt, bake until crispy.

Lunch:
- **Chicken Caesar Salad**
    - o Grilled chicken over romaine with homemade Caesar dressing (using Greek yogurt) and parmesan.

Snack:
- **Dark Chocolate Covered Nuts**
    - o Nuts coated with sugar-free dark chocolate.

Dinner:
- **Stuffed Acorn Squash**
    - o Roasted acorn squash stuffed with quinoa, cranberries, nuts, and herbs.

Day 7
Breakfast:
- **Savory Oatmeal**

o Cook rolled oats in water, topped with avocado, a fried egg, and hot sauce.

Snack:
- **Fruit and Nut Bar**
  - o Homemade bars made from dates, nuts, and seeds, blended and pressed into a pan.

Lunch:
- **Quinoa and Black Bean Bowl**
  - o Quinoa topped with black beans, corn, diced tomatoes, and avocado.

Snack:
- **Cherry Tomatoes and Mozzarella**
  - o Cherry tomatoes drizzled with balsamic vinegar and paired with mozzarella balls.

Dinner:
- **Eggplant Lasagna**
  - o Slices of roasted eggplant layered with marinara sauce and ricotta cheese, baked until bubbly.

Sugar-Free Snack Ideas
1. **Energy Balls**
   - o Blend oats, nut butter, honey (or dates), and add-ins like coconut or chocolate chips.
2. **Veggie Chips**
   - o Slice root vegetables thinly, season, and bake until crispy.
3. **Roasted Nuts**
   - o Season mixed nuts with herbs or spices and roast.

4. **Homemade Trail Mix**
   - o Combine nuts, seeds, and unsweetened dried fruits.

Sugar-Free Dessert Options

1. **Baking with Natural Sweeteners**
   - o Substitute refined sugar with mashed bananas, unsweetened applesauce, or dates in recipes.
2. **Coconut Macaroons**
   - o Made with unsweetened shredded coconut, egg whites, and a natural sweetener.
3. **Chia Seed Pudding**
   - o Sweetened with vanilla extract or pureed fruits, topped with berries.
4. **Frozen Banana Bites**
   - o Banana slices dipped in dark chocolate and frozen.

Tips for Cooking with Low-Glycemic Index Foods

1. **Choose Whole Foods**
   - o Opt for unprocessed grains (quinoa, brown rice) over refined grains (white rice, white bread).
2. **Incorporate More Fiber**
   - o Add fiber-rich foods like beans, legumes, and vegetables to meals.
3. **Balance Your Meals**
   - o Combine proteins, fats, and low-glycemic carbs to stabilize blood sugar.
4. **Limit Processed Foods**
   - o Read labels and choose products with minimal ingredients and no added sugars.

5. **Experiment with Spices**
   o Use spices to enhance flavor without the need for sugar or sauces.

Following this meal plan and tips can help you transition into a sugar free lifestyle while enjoying delicious meals and snacks. Adjust portion sizes according to your individual needs and preferences!

Navigating social situations, especially those involving food, can be challenging for anyone looking to reduce sugar intake. Whether it's a party, a birthday celebration, or a holiday feast, the temptation to indulge can be overwhelming. Here are some detailed strategies and ideas for managing these scenarios without succumbing to sugar binges.

Handling Parties, Birthdays, and Holidays

1. **Plan Ahead:**

    o **Communicate Your Goals:** Let your friends or family know about your dietary preferences ahead of time. This not only sets the tone for your choices but also encourages their support.

    o **Bring Your Own Dish:** If it's

appropriate, offer to bring a healthy dish. This ensures you have something compliant with your goals and introduces others to delicious alternatives. Think of sugar-free desserts, veggie platters with hummus, or protein-rich snacks.

2. **Mindful Eating:**

   o **Survey the Buffet:** Before diving in, take a moment to look over all the options available. This helps you make conscious decisions about what you really want to eat.

   o **Portion Control:** Choose smaller portions or share dishes with a friend. This way, you can enjoy a taste without overindulging.

3. **Stay Hydrated:**

   o **Drink Water:** Often, we mistake thirst for hunger. Keep a glass of water in hand to help manage cravings and prevent overeating.

   o **Choose Sparkling Water or Herbal Tea:** These can be satisfying alternatives to sugary drinks, allowing you to enjoy the social atmosphere without added sugar.

4. Focus on Connections, Not Just Food:

- o **Engage in Conversations:** Shift your focus from food to socializing. Participate in games, dance, or chat with others to keep your mind off eating.

- o **Practice Gratitude:** Remind yourself of the reasons for attending. Focusing on relationships can diminish the urge to snack mindlessly.

Dealing with Peer Pressure: Saying No Without Guilt

1. Prepare Your Responses:

- o **Use Simple Phrases:** Have a few go-to responses ready, such as "I'm focusing on my health right now," or "I'm not hungry, but thank you!" This can make it easier to decline without feeling awkward.

- o **Be Firm Yet Polite:** It's okay to be assertive about your choices. A simple, "No, thank you, I'm good!"

can effectively convey your stance without further discussion.

2. **Set Boundaries:**

    o   **Plan Your Indulgences:** Decide in advance which events are worth a treat and stick to your plan. Allow yourself occasional splurges to feel less deprived.

    o   **Avoid the "All or Nothing" Mentality:** A small bite of cake at a birthday celebration doesn't have to derail your efforts. One small taste can satisfy a craving without leading to a binge.

3. **Surround Yourself with Support:**

    o   **Find Like-Minded Friends:** Seek out friends or acquaintances who share your health goals. They can provide encouragement and help you navigate social pressures together.

    o   **Encourage Others:** Sometimes, sharing your reasons for cutting back on sugar can inspire those around you to join in.

Sugar Detox on the Go: What to Order at Restaurants and Cafes

1. **Choose Wisely:**

   o **Opt for Whole Foods**: Look for meals centered around whole, unprocessed foods. Salads with protein (grilled chicken, tofu, or beans) and plenty of veggies are excellent choices.

   o **Ask for Modifications:** Don't hesitate to ask for changes, like dressing on the side or skipping sweet sauces. Most restaurants are willing to accommodate requests.

2. **Satisfy Your Sweet Tooth Healthily:**

   o **Fresh Fruit or Sorbet:** If you want dessert, consider ordering fresh fruit or a scoop of sorbet instead of cake or pastries.

   o **Dark Chocolate:** If available, dark chocolate (70% cocoa or higher) can be a satisfying treat that is lower in sugar.

3. **Beverage Choices:**

   o **Skip Sugary Drinks:** Choose water, unsweetened iced tea, or black coffee instead of sodas or sweetened beverages.

   o **Alcohol Considerations:** If you drink

alcohol, opt for spirits with soda water and a splash of lemon or lime, avoiding sugary mixers.

Preparing Your Environment: Avoiding Temptations at Home and Work

1. **Stock Up on Healthy Options.**

    o **Keep Healthy Snacks Accessible:** Fill your pantry with nuts, seeds, dried fruits (unsweetened), and fresh fruits. Having nutritious snacks on hand reduces the temptation to reach for sugary options.

    o **Meal Prep:** Preparing healthy meals in advance can help you avoid the last-minute temptation to order takeout or grab unhealthy snacks.

2. **Clear Out Temptations:**

    o **Minimize Sugar in the Home:** If possible, reduce or eliminate sugary snacks from your home. Out of sight can help keep them out of mind.

    o **Create a "Treat" Zone:** If you have kids or family members who enjoy sweets, designate a specific spot for treats that's less accessible to you.

3. **Mindful Workspace Setup:**

o **Healthy Office Snacks:** Bring in your own healthy snacks to keep at your desk. This not only helps you but also can encourage colleagues to choose healthier options.

o **Avoid the Break Room:** If the break room is a frequent temptation, try to minimize time spent there or bring healthy alternatives when others are indulging.

Additional Tips for Success

1. **Celebrate Small Wins:** Acknowledge your successes in avoiding sugar, whether it's passing on dessert or choosing healthy options at a restaurant. Celebrating small victories can motivate you to keep going.

2. **Practice Self-Compassion:** If you do indulge, don't beat yourself up. Instead, reflect on what led to that choice and how you can prepare for future situations.

3. **Continuous Learning:** Educate yourself about nutrition and sugar's effects on the body. The more informed you are, the easier it becomes to make choices aligned with your health goals.

By employing these strategies, you can successfully navigate social situations while minimizing sugar consumption, making it easier to stick to your health goals and enjoy your time with others.

The Mind–Body Connection: Staying Motivated and Consistent During a Sugar Detox

When working toward breaking free from sugar cravings, it's important to align both physical and mental health.

A well-balanced strategy that incorporates exercise, hydration, sleep, stress management, and emotional tools will help you stay motivated and consistent.

Below is a deeper exploration of these concepts with actionable advice to keep you on track.

---

1. The Role of Exercise in Managing Sugar Cravings

Physical movement doesn't just benefit your body—it can directly influence your brain and curb cravings.

- **How Exercise Reduces Sugar Cravings:**

    o Physical activity releases endorphins and dopamine, the same chemicals that sugar triggers in your brain, creating a natural high.

    o Exercise stabilizes blood sugar levels, reducing sudden dips that often lead to cravings.

    o It helps regulate insulin sensitivity, promoting a balanced appetite.

- **Best Types of Exercise for a Sugar Detox:**

    o Aerobic exercises (like walking, running, or swimming) can help reduce stress, which in turn

    minimizes emotional cravings.

    o Strength training stabilizes glucose levels and supports metabolism.

    o Yoga and Pilates improve body awareness and mindfulness, which helps in resisting mindless eating.

    o Short bursts of exercise (like 5–10 minutes of jumping jacks or a quick jog) are great during moments of intense cravings.

- Tip: Schedule consistent, enjoyable activities (like dancing or group classes) to make exercise a habit and keep motivation high.

---

2. Importance of Hydration and Balanced Electrolytes

Many times, sugar cravings are mistaken signals for dehydration or electrolyte imbalances. Staying hydrated can prevent these cravings and help your body function optimally during detox.

- **How Hydration Reduces Cravings:**

    o Water regulates blood sugar and flushes toxins from the body.

    o It prevents fatigue and brain fog, which are common withdrawal symptoms during detox.

    o Drinking water can fill your stomach, tricking your brain into feeling satiated.

- **Electrolyte Imbalance and Cravings:**

    o When cutting out sugar, you may experience low energy levels, partly due to electrolyte imbalances (low sodium, potassium, or magnesium).

o   Without balanced electrolytes, your body might mistake the need for minerals as sugar cravings.

- **How to Stay Hydrated:**

    o   Aim for 8-10 glasses of water daily, or more if you're exercising.

    o   Add a pinch of sea salt and a squeeze of lemon to water for electrolytes.

    o   Consume foods like coconut water, leafy greens, bananas, and avocados to replenish potassium and magnesium levels.

    o   Keep a water bottle with you at all times and sip throughout the day to avoid dehydration.

---

3. Sleep and Stress Management for Better Hormonal Balance

Lack of sleep and unmanaged stress can sabotage your detox efforts by disrupting hormones that control appetite and cravings.

- **The Hormonal Connection:**

  - o Sleep deprivation causes an increase in ghrelin (the hunger hormone) and a drop in leptin (the hormone that signals fullness). This imbalance triggers sugar cravings.

  - o Stress releases cortisol, which prompts your body to crave quick sources of energy (like sugar) for a temporary mood boost.

  - o Poor sleep and stress impair insulin sensitivity, making it harder to stabilize blood sugar.

- **Tips to Improve Sleep During Detox:**

  - o Create a wind-down routine (like reading or listening to soothing music) to signal your brain it's time to sleep.

  - o Avoid caffeine, sugar, and screen time 2-3 hours before bedtime.

  - o Use magnesium supplements or herbal teas (like chamomile or lavender) to relax your body.

- **Stress Management Strategies:**

    o   Practice breathing exercises (like box breathing: inhale 4 seconds, hold 4 seconds, exhale 4 seconds).

    o   Use mindfulness techniques such as meditation, journaling, or body scans to become aware of emotional triggers for sugar cravings.

    o   Engage in stress-relieving activities like yoga, nature walks, or art therapy.

---

4. Visualization Techniques to Maintain Motivation

o

Visualization is a powerful tool that taps into the mind-body connection and strengthens motivation.

- **How Visualization Helps:**

    o   When you visualize your goals clearly, your brain becomes more focused on achieving them.

    o   Imagining yourself succeeding in your sugar detox journey increases emotional resilience and reinforces your commitment.

o   Visualization can reduce stress and anxiety by helping you stay positive during challenging moments.

- **How to Use Visualization Daily:**

    o   **Morning practice:** Spend 5 minutes visualizing yourself feeling energetic, healthy, and free from cravings. Imagine how good it feels to achieve your goal.

    o   **Craving control:** When cravings hit, visualize your future self choosing a healthy snack instead or drinking water to resist the

    temptation.

    o   Create a vision board with images and affirmations related to your detox goals (e.g., pictures of healthy foods, fitness activities, or inspiring quotes).

---

4. Building a Support System: Accountability Buddies or Groups

It's hard to go through a sugar detox alone. Accountability partners or support groups can boost motivation, keep you focused, and offer valuable advice.

- **Why Accountability Works:**

  - Having someone to check in with helps you stay committed and consistent.

  - Sharing struggles and victories with others reinforces positive behavior and provides encouragement.

  - You're less likely to relapse when you know someone is counting on you to follow through.

- **Ways to Build a Support System:**

  - **Find an accountability buddy:** A friend, family member, or co-worker who shares your detox goals. Schedule regular check-ins via text or phone calls.

  - **Join online groups:** Look for Facebook groups, Reddit communities, or local meetups focused on health, sugar detox, or fitness. Engage actively to stay motivated and learn new tips.

  - **Use habit-tracking apps with**

friends: Apps like Habitica or MyFitnessPal allow you to track progress and share updates with others, creating friendly competition.

Bonus: Creating a Holistic Routine to Stay Consistent

Creating a structured daily routine that combines these mind-body strategies will help you maintain consistency and avoid burnout. Here's an example:

Morning:
- Hydrate first thing (add lemon and salt for electrolytes).
- Spend 5 minutes visualizing your detox success and setting a positive intention for the day.
- Exercise for 20-30 minutes to boost your mood and energy.

Afternoon:
- Eat a balanced lunch with healthy proteins, fats, and fiber to avoid afternoon sugar cravings.
- Take a short walk after meals to support digestion and blood sugar levels.
- Check in with your accountability buddy or support group to share progress.

Evening:

- Unwind with a relaxation routine (breathing exercises, meditation, or reading).

- Review your progress journal or log into your tracking app to reflect on wins and challenges.

- Aim for 7–8 hours of quality sleep by going to bed at a consistent time.

Conclusion: Strengthening the Mind-Body Connection for Long-Term Success

The journey to break free from sugar isn't just about willpower—it requires mindful strategies that nurture both your body and mind. By integrating exercise, hydration, sleep hygiene, stress management, visualization, and social support into your routine, you'll build a sustainable system that keeps you motivated and consistent.

With these tools, you'll be well-prepared to overcome cravings, maintain energy levels, and experience the full benefits of a sugar-free lifestyle—one step at a time.

Sugar Alternatives: What Works and What Doesn't

Cutting out sugar can be tough, but using sugar alternatives can help ease the transition. However, **not all substitutes are created equal**—some may affect cravings, digestion, or long-term health. In this section, we'll explore **artificial sweeteners, natural alternatives, and the dos and don'ts** of using them to stay on track with your sugar detox goals.

---

1. Artificial Sweeteners: Pros, Cons, and Controversies

Artificial sweeteners are synthetic substitutes that mimic sugar's sweetness without adding calories. They are widely used in **diet sodas, sugar-free snacks, and "low-calorie" products**, but they remain controversial for their potential health risks.

Examples of Common Artificial Sweeteners:

- **Aspartame** (Equal, NutraSweet)
- **Sucralose** (Splenda)
- **Saccharin** (Sweet'N Low)
- **Acesulfame-K** (often found in sugar-free gums and soft drinks)

Pros:

- **Zero or very low calories**: Useful for those trying to manage weight.
- **Doesn't raise blood sugar**: Beneficial for people with diabetes.
- **Widely available**: Found in many products marketed as "sugar-free."

Cons:

- **May disrupt gut health**: Some artificial sweeteners (e.g., sucralose) have been shown to negatively affect the **gut microbiome**.

- **Potential to trigger cravings**: These sweeteners can **confuse the brain** into expecting calories, which may lead to increased cravings for sweet foods.

- **Health concerns**: Studies link high consumption of some sweeteners to **metabolic disorders** and other health risks, although findings are mixed.

- **Aftertaste**: Many artificial sweeteners have a distinct, chemical aftertaste that some people dislike.

Verdict:

Artificial sweeteners can be a **short-term aid**, especially for those trying to quit sugary drinks or snacks. However, it's wise to **limit long-term use**, as they may perpetuate cravings and pose health concerns.

---

2. Natural Alternatives: Stevia, Monk Fruit, Coconut Sugar, Honey

Natural sugar substitutes are often marketed as **healthier alternatives**. While they come from plants or natural sources, they still require careful use to avoid triggering cravings or blood sugar spikes.

Stevia:

- **Made from**: The leaves of the stevia plant.
- **Sweetness**: 200-300 times sweeter than

sugar, but with no calories.

- **Pros**: Doesn't spike blood sugar or insulin levels.
- **Cons**: Some people find it has a **bitter aftertaste**. Highly processed forms may contain additives.
- **Best Use**: Add to beverages like tea or coffee or use in baking (but in very small amounts due to its sweetness).

Monk Fruit:

- **Made from**: A fruit native to Southeast Asia.
- **Sweetness**: 150-200 times sweeter than sugar, but with zero calories.
- **Pros**: Won't raise blood sugar and has **antioxidant properties**.
- **Cons**: Pure monk fruit is expensive, and many products contain **fillers like erythritol** (a sugar alcohol).
- **Best Use**: Works well in baking, smoothies, and hot beverages.

Coconut Sugar:

- **Made from**: The sap of the coconut palm.
- **Sweetness**: Similar to white sugar but with a **caramel-like flavor**.
- **Pros**: Contains small amounts of minerals and has a **lower glycemic index** than

refined sugar.

- **Cons**: It's still sugar and can cause **blood sugar spikes** if consumed in excess.
- **Best Use**: Use sparingly in baking or cooking where a caramel flavor is desired.

Honey:

- **Made by**: Bees from flower nectar.
- **Sweetness**: Sweeter than sugar, with more flavor complexity.
- **Pros**: Contains **antioxidants, vitamins, and antibacterial properties**.
- **Cons**: Honey can **spike blood sugar** and add calories if used in excess.
- **Best Use**: A great addition to tea, yogurt, or homemade salad dressings—but in small amounts.

---

3. Using Sugar Substitutes Wisely to Avoid Triggering Cravings

While sugar alternatives can make your detox easier, **misusing them might keep you trapped in a craving cycle**. Here are some strategies to use them effectively:

Tips for Using Sugar Substitutes Wisely:

1. **Limit Frequency and Amount**: Even zero-calorie sweeteners can **keep your taste buds hooked on sweetness**. Use

them sparingly as an occasional treat, rather than a daily habit.

2. **Combine with Protein or Fiber**: Eating sugar substitutes with protein or fiber can **stabilize blood sugar levels** and reduce the risk of cravings.

3. **Retrain Your Palate**: Over time, **reduce your reliance on sweet tastes** by gradually using less and less of these alternatives. Focus on enjoying the **natural sweetness of fruits** instead.

4. **Track Your Cravings**: If you notice that sweeteners are **triggering sugar cravings**, consider cutting them out for a few weeks to break the pattern.

5. **Avoid Overindulgence**: Just because a product is sugar-free doesn't mean it's **healthy**—read labels to check for added fats, artificial chemicals, or hidden sugars.

---

4. Substitutes to Avoid for Long-Term Success

Some substitutes, although marketed as healthy, **may not support your detox journey**. Certain options can still cause **blood sugar spikes**, trigger cravings, or come with health risks.

Agave Syrup:

- **Why to Avoid**: It's often marketed as a low-glycemic sweetener, but it contains **high amounts of fructose**, which can increase the risk of **insulin resistance** and liver problems.
- **Alternative**: Opt for small amounts of **honey or coconut sugar** if you need a natural sweetener.

Erythritol and Other Sugar Alcohols:

- **Why to Avoid**: While sugar alcohols (like erythritol, xylitol, or maltitol) have fewer calories than sugar, they can cause **bloating, gas, and digestive discomfort** in some people.
- **Alternative**: If sugar alcohols work for you, **use in small quantities**. Otherwise, **monk fruit or stevia** might be better options.

Fruit Juices:

- **Why to Avoid**: Even though they are natural, **fruit juices are high in fructose** and lack the fiber of whole fruits. This makes them more likely to cause **blood sugar spikes**.
- **Alternative**: Eat **whole fruits** instead to get natural sweetness along with fiber,

vitamins, and minerals.

Flavored Syrups and Sweetened Condiments:

- **Why to Avoid**: Many flavored syrups (like maple-flavored syrup or sugar-free syrups) contain **artificial chemicals, high-fructose corn syrup, or hidden sugars.**
- **Alternative**: If you need flavor, use a **small drizzle of pure honey** or add natural sweetness with **vanilla extract or cinnamon.**

---

5. Conclusion: Choosing the Right Sugar Alternatives for Your Journey

Not all sugar substitutes are equal when it comes to **supporting long-term success**. While some natural alternatives like **stevia, monk fruit, or coconut sugar** can be helpful tools, others like **agave syrup or fruit juice** might derail your efforts by spiking blood sugar or triggering cravings. The key is to **use alternatives wisely, in moderation, and gradually reduce your dependence on sweetness** over time.

Instead of focusing solely on finding the perfect sweetener, aim to **retrain your palate** and savor the natural sweetness found in whole foods like fruits, nuts, and vegetables. With a mindful approach, you'll not only **reduce cravings** but also experience the **freedom and energy** that comes with living a sugar-free lifestyle.

10 RELAPSING

Relapse and Getting Back on Track
Relapses are a natural part of the process when you're working to overcome sugar addiction or create healthier habits. The key isn't to avoid setbacks entirely (because they *will* happen), but to **learn from them and keep moving forward**. By developing resilience, being flexible with yourself, and reinforcing healthy routines, you can prevent a minor slip-up from becoming a full-blown return to old habits. In this section, we'll explore how to **handle relapses, build emotional resilience, and maintain a sustainable lifestyle**.

1. **Why Relapses are Normal and How to Handle Them**

Relapses are common because **breaking habits connected to cravings is challenging**—especially when emotions, stress, or social situations come into play. It's important to understand that **slipping up doesn't mean failure**. In fact, experiencing a relapse can teach you valuable lessons about what triggers your cravings and what strategies you need to strengthen.

Why Relapses Happen:

- **Biological urges**: Sugar causes dopamine surges in the brain, creating a reward cycle that can be difficult to break.

- **Emotional triggers**: Stress, boredom, anxiety, or loneliness can make you turn to sugar for comfort.

- **Social pressure**: Celebrations, holidays, or peer pressure can lead to unintentional indulgence.

- **Exhaustion or burnout**: Lack of sleep or mental fatigue makes it harder to resist cravings.

How to Handle a Relapse:

1. **Don't Punish Yourself**: Self-criticism after a relapse often leads to a vicious cycle of guilt and further indulgence. Instead, **accept**

it as part of the process and move forward.

2. **Pause and Reflect**: Ask yourself what caused the relapse. **Was it emotional? Social? Physical exhaustion?** Identifying the root cause will help you prevent similar situations in the future.

3. **Use it as Feedback**: A relapse isn't failure—it's information. **Journal or reflect on what you learned** so you can adjust your approach.

4. **Get Back on Track Immediately**: Don't wait for tomorrow or next Monday—**the next healthy choice is your comeback**. Make your next meal or snack sugar-free to regain momentum.

2. Building Resilience: Learning from Setbacks

Resilience is the ability to **bounce back quickly** after a setback and stay committed to your long-term goals. Learning to **handle challenges with self-compassion and patience** will make it easier to stay on track, even when the road isn't smooth.

How to Build Resilience After a Setback:

- **Reframe Setbacks as Part of the Process**: Remind yourself that **progress isn't**

linear—there will always be ups and downs. Every time you recover from a relapse, you strengthen your ability to persevere.

- **Identify Patterns**: Look for **triggers or weak moments**. Do cravings spike when you're stressed? Do social events tempt you? Identifying these patterns helps you **prepare in advance** for future challenges.

- **Set Small Recovery Goals**: Focus on **one healthy action at a time** rather than overwhelming yourself with unrealistic expectations (e.g., "I'll eat only whole foods forever"). If you slip, **drink a glass of water**, go for a walk, or eat a healthy meal to build momentum.

- **Celebrate Your Wins**: Recognize and **celebrate small victories**—like choosing water over soda or saying no to dessert at a party. These wins keep you motivated.

The Power of Self-Compassion:

Studies show that **self-compassion helps people stick to their goals**. Instead of criticizing yourself after a setback, say, "This is part of the journey. I'm learning, and I'll do better next time." **Forgiveness fosters resilience**, making it easier to stay consistent in the long run.

- ### 3. Developing a Flexible Approach: Creating Space for Occasional Treats

A rigid, all-or-nothing approach to cutting sugar can lead to burnout and increase the risk of bingeing after a minor slip. Instead, a **flexible approach allows you to enjoy occasional treats in a mindful way**, without falling back into old patterns.

Why Flexibility Matters:

- **Psychological relief**: When you know you can have the occasional treat, it **removes the feeling of deprivation**, making it easier to resist daily temptations.

- **Long-term sustainability**: A flexible approach ensures that **healthy eating becomes a lifestyle** rather than a short-term diet.

- **Improves social experiences**: Flexibility allows you to enjoy **celebrations and gatherings** without guilt, fostering a healthy relationship with food.

How to Create Space for Treats:

- **Plan Ahead**: If you know you'll have dessert at a special occasion, **make it a conscious choice** and balance the rest of your meals around it.

- **Savor Mindfully**: Instead of mindlessly indulging, **slow down** and enjoy each bite. This can reduce the desire to overeat and help you feel satisfied.

- **Use the 80/20 Rule**: Aim to **eat healthily 80% of the time**, leaving room for treats 20% of the time. This helps keep things realistic without compromising your progress.

- **Set Personal Boundaries**: Be clear with yourself—**what counts as a reasonable treat?** A slice of cake at a party? A latte with honey on weekends? Decide in advance to avoid slipping into a pattern of frequent indulgence.

---

3. Reinforcing Healthy Habits so Sugar Doesn't Sneak Back In

To stay sugar-free for the long haul, it's essential to **reinforce new habits and be mindful of situations where sugar might creep back into your**

diet. Building sustainable habits ensures you **maintain control** without feeling constantly deprived or stressed.

Tips for Reinforcing Healthy Habits:

1. **Stock Your Kitchen with Healthy Alternatives**: Keep **fresh fruits, nuts, yogurt, and herbal teas** on hand so you're not tempted by sugary snacks.

2. **Stay Consistent with Meal Planning**: Plan meals in advance to avoid relying on **processed convenience foods**, which often contain hidden sugars.

3. **Be Aware of Hidden Sugars**: Carefully read food labels—**sugar sneaks into items** like sauces, salad dressings, and granola bars. Look for terms like "syrup," "malt," or "fructose."

4. **Develop Non-Food Rewards**: Celebrate your progress with **non-food rewards** like a new book, a relaxing bath, or a night out with friends. This helps you avoid using treats as a reward system.

5. **Check In with Yourself Regularly**: Reflect weekly or monthly on how you're feeling. Are cravings creeping back? Are you starting to rely on sugar substitutes? **Adjust your strategies as needed** to stay on track.

6. Example: How to Get Back on Track After a Relapse

Scenario: You've been sugar-free for three weeks, but you gave in to a cupcake at a work party. Now you feel guilty and tempted to give up.

Step 1: **Pause and Reflect**: Recognize that this is normal. "It's just one cupcake, not a disaster." Ask yourself what caused the slip—**were you stressed or caught off-guard by the temptation?**

Step 2: **Take Immediate Action**: Drink a glass of water and **choose a healthy dinner** that aligns with your detox plan (like a salad with lean protein). This helps re-establish momentum.

Step 3: **Journal or Reflect**: Write about the situation in a journal—what can you do differently next time? **Bring awareness** to the trigger, so you're prepared in future situations.

Step 4: **Move On**: Remember, progress isn't about being perfect. **Focus on the next healthy decision**, and don't dwell on the relapse.

6. Conclusion: Relapse is Part of Progress

Relapse is not a sign of failure—it's a **normal part of change**. Each time you experience a setback and recover from it, you **build resilience** and get stronger. By staying flexible, learning from your experiences, and reinforcing healthy habits, you'll gain more control over sugar cravings and maintain progress for the long term.

The key is to **embrace the journey, not just the destination**. Mistakes and detours are part of the process, but with self-compassion, smart strategies, and a flexible mindset, you'll find your way back to balance every time.

Success stories and testimonials
Hearing about real people who have successfully transformed their lives by **breaking free from sugar addiction** can be incredibly inspiring. These stories offer **motivation, practical advice, and hope**, showing that it's possible to overcome cravings, build healthy habits, and feel better physically and mentally. Additionally, insights from health experts and nutritionists provide **evidence-based guidance** that reinforces the benefits of cutting sugar.

---

1. **Real-life case studies: stories of people who quit sugar and thrived**

Here are a few types of success stories you could feature. These stories **humanize the sugar detox process**, showing that even with setbacks, people can persevere and enjoy profound benefits.

Case study 1: from chronic fatigue to vibrant energy

- **Background**: Sarah, a 40-year-old mother of two, struggled with fatigue, brain fog, and afternoon crashes. She relied on sugary coffee drinks and snacks throughout the day to get through.

- **Journey**: after starting a **30-day sugar detox**, Sarah experienced headaches and cravings in the first week but stuck to her plan. She replaced sugary snacks with **fruit, nuts, and protein-rich foods.**

- **Results**: by the end of the detox, Sarah reported **stable energy levels, fewer mood swings**, and improved focus. She now uses **meal prepping and journaling** to stay consistent and indulges in occasional treats mindfully.

- **Key takeaway**: learning to recognize sugar as a trigger for fatigue was life-changing for Sarah. She says, "I never realized how much sugar was draining me. Now i feel energized, and I don't need sugar to get through the day."

Case study 2: overcoming emotional eating with a mindful approach

- **Background**: Jason, a 32-year-old sales executive, turned to **sweets to cope with stress and emotional exhaustion** from his high-pressure job. His sugar consumption caused **weight gain and anxiety**.

- **Journey**: with the help of a therapist, Jason began practicing **mindful eating** and journaling his triggers. He gradually replaced sugary comfort foods with **tea, dark chocolate, and fresh fruit.**

- **Results**: over six months, Jason lost 15 pounds, improved his sleep, and reduced his anxiety. His biggest achievement was learning to **manage stress without relying on sugar**.

- **Key takeaway**: Jason says, "the breakthrough for me was learning that cravings are often emotional, not physical. Now, instead of grabbing candy, i take a walk or call a friend."

Case study 3: beating sugar to improve mental health

- **Background**: Emma, 28, struggled with **depression and anxiety**, which worsened with her reliance on sugary comfort foods like pastries and ice cream.

- **Journey**: after consulting with a nutritionist, Emma embarked on a **gradual sugar detox**, replacing sweets with nutrient-dense foods like **omega-3-rich salmon and leafy greens**. She also practiced **meditation** to cope with stress.

- **Results**: Emma noticed a significant **improvement in her mood** after two months. Her anxiety lessened, and her depressive episodes became less frequent.

- **Key takeaway**: Emma says, "I didn't realize how much sugar was contributing to my mental health struggles. Cutting it out gave me clarity and emotional stability I didn't think was possible."

---

2. **Expert insights: interviews with health professionals and coaches**

Including advice from **nutritionists, health coaches, and fitness trainers** adds credibility to the book. These experts can offer **practical tips, debunk myths**, and highlight the **scientific benefits** of quitting sugar.
Interview with a nutritionist: "breaking the cycle of cravings"

- **Key topic**: why sugar cravings happen and how to overcome them

- **Advice**: "it's important to recognize that **sugar cravings are linked to blood sugar imbalances**. One way to stabilize your levels is to include **protein and healthy fats** in every meal. This keeps you fuller longer and reduces sugar cravings."

- **Additional tip**: "don't aim for perfection. Plan for **small indulgences**, and focus on building a sustainable lifestyle."

Fitness coach: "how exercise helps you beat cravings"

- **Key topic**: how physical activity affects sugar withdrawal and cravings

- **Advice**: "exercise boosts the release of **endorphins** and helps regulate insulin levels, both of which reduce the urge to reach for sugary foods. Even 30 minutes of walking or yoga can have a significant impact."

- **Additional tip**: "pair exercise with a sugar detox. When you feel the benefits—like more energy—it's easier to stay motivated."

Mental health expert: "the emotional side of sugar addiction"

- **Key topic**: how emotional triggers affect sugar cravings and what to do about it

- **Advice**: "sugar often becomes a coping mechanism for **emotional stress**, so it's essential to address those emotions directly. **Journaling, meditation, and therapy** can all help When you deal with the root cause, the cravings naturally lessen."

- **Additional tip**: "reward yourself with **non-food activities**, like going for a massage or watching a movie, to avoid the trap of emotional eating."

---

3. Motivational tips from individuals who beat sugar addiction

These **first-hand tips** from people who've succeeded in eliminating sugar can offer actionable advice and inspire others to stay on track.

- **"it's okay to slip up."**
  "the biggest lesson i learned is that **perfection isn't the goal**—progress is. If you relapse, just get back on track with your

next meal. Don't wait for Monday or a new month. Every meal is a chance to start fresh."

- **"find healthier comfort foods."**
  "i used to rely on ice cream when i was stressed, but now i make a habit of drinking **herbal tea** or having a piece of **dark chocolate**. It satisfies the craving without derailing my progress."

- **"meal prep makes all the difference."**
  "the turning point for me was when i started **prepping healthy snacks** ahead of time. Having easy options like **carrot**

  sticks, boiled eggs, or hummus made it easier to resist sugary temptations."
- **"accountability is key."**

  "I joined a **facebook group** for people on the same detox journey, and it kept me going. Just knowing that others were struggling and succeeding made a huge difference."

4. **How these success stories inspire and motivate**

Reading about others' journeys and expert advice makes the sugar detox process feel **achievable and real**. Success stories offer:

- **Validation**: it's normal to struggle with cravings, relapses, and setbacks.

- **Hope**: even small steps can lead to **life-changing results**.

- **Practical inspiration**: real-world strategies from people who've done it offer **new ways to stay on track**.

These stories remind readers that **they're not alone** and that success isn't about perfection—it's about **making progress, one step at a time**.

---

5. Conclusion: your story could be next
The inspiring testimonials and expert advice throughout this section demonstrate that **transforming your life by quitting sugar is possible**—no matter where you're starting from. You might experience **cravings, challenges, and even relapses**, but with the right tools and mindset, you can push through.
In time, your own journey could become an inspiration to others. By embracing progress over perfection, using the strategies that work for you, and staying connected to a supportive community, you'll be able to create **a healthier, happier life** without sugar. Who knows—your story could be the next success story shared to inspire someone

else on their journey!

12 CONCLUSION

Conclusion: your new sweet life
Congratulations! You've made it to the end of this journey, and whether you're just starting or well on your way, **every step forward is something to celebrate**. Choosing to break free from sugar isn't just about saying goodbye to sweets—it's about embracing **a healthier, more vibrant life**. In this final chapter, let's explore how to celebrate your progress, maintain momentum, and **make a sugar-free lifestyle sustainable and rewarding** for the long haul.

1. **Celebrating your progress and personal wins**

Recognizing the small victories along the way is crucial to **staying motivated**. Your journey hasn't been about perfection—it's been about progress, resilience, and commitment to taking care of yourself.

What progress looks like:

- **Cravings feel more manageable**. You've learned how to identify triggers and respond with healthier choices.

- **You bounce back faster** from slip-ups. Instead of spiraling into guilt after indulging, you refocus on your goals.

  Healthier habits feel natural. Maybe you've replaced soda with sparkling water or enjoy fruit instead of desserts—small changes that add up.

Ways to celebrate your wins:

- **Non-food rewards**: treat yourself to a massage, a new book, or a day outdoors.

- **Reflect on milestones**: write in a journal about how your energy, mood, or physical health has improved.

- **Create a visual progress tracker**: mark off sugar-free days on a calendar or use an app to log your wins.

- **Share your story**: sharing your progress with friends, family, or on social media can inspire others to follow your lead and give you a sense of accomplishment.

---

2. How your body, mind, and energy improve without sugar

As you've reduced your sugar intake, you've probably started noticing significant changes in your **physical, mental, and emotional well-being**. The improvements extend far beyond

 losing weight—they affect **how you feel and function every day**.

Physical benefits:

- **Stable energy levels**: no more crashing in the afternoon. Your energy is steady throughout the day, thanks to balanced blood sugar levels.

- **Improved digestion**: less bloating, fewer cravings, and a healthier gut—free from sugary snacks that disrupt your digestive system.

- **Clearer skin**: many people find that reducing sugar reduces acne, redness, or inflammation.

- **Better sleep**: without sugar highs and lows disrupting your hormones, you sleep more soundly and wake up refreshed.

Mental and emotional benefits:

- **Mental clarity and focus**: sugar fogs the brain, but cutting it out sharpens your thinking and enhances focus.

- **Reduced mood swings**: with sugar no longer dictating your mood, you feel calmer, more balanced, and in control.

- **Better emotional regulation**: instead of reaching for sugar when stressed, you've developed healthier ways to manage emotions.

How your relationships improve:

- **More present and engaged**: with stable

energy and fewer mood swings, you're more engaged in relationships and conversations.

- **Positive ripple effect**: your healthy habits may have inspired family and friends to make changes, creating a healthier environment for everyone.

---

3. Making the sugar-free lifestyle sustainable

The key to long-term success is to **find joy in your new habits** and build a lifestyle that works for you. Sustainability isn't about deprivation—it's about **balance, flexibility, and learning to enjoy food in a new way**.
Tips for a sustainable sugar-free lifestyle:

1. **Focus on whole foods**: the more you rely on whole, unprocessed foods, the easier it is to avoid hidden sugars.

2. **Plan for treats**: create space for occasional indulgences so you don't feel deprived. Plan them mindfully—savoring a dessert at a birthday party or enjoying honey in your tea on weekends.

3. **Rotate new recipes**: keep things exciting by trying **new sugar-free recipes** regularly. Discovering delicious, healthy alternatives will make your journey enjoyable.

4. **Stay aware of sneaky sugars**: always read labels. Many "health" foods hide

    sugar under names like **agave nectar, malt syrup, or fructose**.

5. **Review and adjust**: every few weeks, check in with yourself—**are you still enjoying your new habits? Are cravings under control?** Make adjustments if needed, so the process stays manageable.

6. **Develop non-food coping strategies**: life will throw challenges your way—stress, boredom, or emotional triggers. **Find other ways to cope**: walk, meditate, journal, or connect with a friend instead of turning to sugar.

Anchor your motivation to long-term goals:

- Visualize **how you'll feel in 1 year** without sugar: more energy, better health, greater self-confidence.

- Remind yourself of **why you started**—whether to improve your health, feel better in your body, or set a good example for your family.
- Stay flexible: allow room for occasional treats, but always return to your **core healthy habits**.

4. Encouraging readers to share their journeys
Your journey is unique and meaningful—and
sharing it can inspire others who are struggling
with sugar addiction. When you tell your story, it
not only reinforces your commitment, but it also
creates a **sense of community and support**.

Why sharing matters:

- **It motivates others**: hearing real-life stories
  makes people feel less alone and more
  hopeful.

- **It holds you accountable**: when you share
  your goals publicly—whether with friends,
  on social media, or in support
  groups—you're more likely to stay
  consistent.

- **It creates a support network**: you'll connect
  with like-minded people who are on a
  similar journey, offering

- encouragement and advice.

Ways to share your journey:

1. **Join online communities**: participate in
   facebook groups or reddit threads
   dedicated to sugar detoxes or healthy
   living.

2. **Start a blog or instagram account**: document your progress, share recipes, and celebrate milestones publicly.

3. **Support a friend or family member**: encourage others by sharing your experiences and **offering to detox together**. Accountability makes the process easier.

4. **Write testimonials**: if you used a specific book, app, or detox program, **write a review** to help others who are just starting out.

5. **Keep a private journal**: even if you don't want to share publicly, **documenting your thoughts and**

    progress helps solidify your new habits.

---

6. **Embrace the journey ahead: a lifestyle, not a destination**

Your sugar detox isn't just a **temporary fix**—it's a step toward a **lifelong transformation**. The goal isn't to be perfect, but to **create a balanced relationship with food and find joy in healthy choices**. You'll continue to learn and grow along the way, and each step brings you closer to a more vibrant, energized, and fulfilling life.

Remember: the occasional slip-up doesn't undo

your progress. **Every healthy choice** counts, and every time you return to your sugar-free habits, you strengthen them. This is your new sweet life—a life where **you're in control**, where food nourishes you without weighing you down, and where you can enjoy the present without relying on sugar.

---

7.   Your journey is just the beginning

There's no finish line—just **ongoing growth, learning, and progress**. Whether you stay completely sugar-free or adopt a flexible approach, the most important thing is that you've reclaimed control over your health. The best part? **Your new sweet life feels better than anything sugar could offer.**

So, take a moment to reflect on how far you've come. Celebrate your wins, share your journey, and keep moving forward. You've got

everything you need to live a life full of **energy, balance, and joy**—without sugar holding you back.

Now, it's time to **write the next chapter of your story.** What will your new sweet life look like from here?

BONUS CONTENT: RESOURCES AND TOOLS

Having the right tools and resources at your fingertips can make your sugar detox journey smoother and more enjoyable. This section offers practical guides, apps, books, podcasts, and templates to help you stay on track, build healthy habits, and remain sugar-free in the long term.

---

1. **Grocery shopping lists**: what to stock up on Transforming your kitchen is a key step to detoxing from sugar. Stock up on wholesome, nutrient-dense foods to avoid the temptation of sugary snacks. This list breaks down essential pantry, fridge, and freezer items, ensuring you're always prepared.

PANTRY STAPLES:

Healthy fats: olive oil, avocado oil, coconut oil,

ghee
Whole grains: oats, quinoa, brown rice, whole-wheat pasta
Nuts & seeds: almonds, walnuts, chia seeds, sunflower seeds, flaxseeds
Natural sweeteners: stevia, monk fruit, raw honey (in moderation)
Protein sources: lentils, beans, chickpeas, canned tuna or salmon
Spices & seasonings: cinnamon, turmeric, cayenne, vanilla extract (no sugar)
Snacks: unsweetened nut butter, roasted chickpeas, popcorn, seaweed snacks
Fridge essentials:
Vegetables: leafy greens, bell peppers, broccoli, zucchini, cauliflower
Fruit: berries, apples, citrus fruits, avocados
Dairy or alternatives: unsweetened yogurt, almond or oat milk
Protein: eggs, tofu, chicken breasts, lean meats, fish

Freezer favorites:

Frozen vegetables: spinach, peas, mixed veggies
Frozen fruit: mango, blueberries, raspberries (great for smoothies)
Pre-cooked meals: homemade soups, stews, or chili
Healthy treats: diy frozen banana pops or homemade energy bites

---

2. Recommended apps, books, and podcasts for

sugar detox support

Staying sugar-free is easier when you're supported by technology and inspiring content. Here are the best apps, books, and podcasts to motivate, track, and guide you throughout your detox journey.

Apps:

Myfitnesspal: track your daily food intake and sugar consumption.
Habitica: turn habit-building into a fun, game-like experience with rewards for sticking to your detox.
Yazio: track calories, meals, and macronutrients while monitoring hidden sugars in foods.
Aloe bud: a gentle app for self-care reminders, including hydration and mindful eating habits.
Zero: track fasting hours (if you're incorporating intermittent fasting) to manage sugar cravings.

Books:

"the case against sugar" by gary taubes: explores how sugar became a staple in our diets and the health consequences it brings.

"bright line eating" by susan peirce thompson: a comprehensive plan to break free from sugar and other processed foods.

"the 21-day sugar detox" by diane sanfilippo: a step-by-step program with recipes and meal plans to help you reset your sugar cravings.

"quit like a woman" by holly whitaker: although primarily about alcohol, the principles of behavior change are applicable to sugar addiction too.

Podcasts.

The model health show: episodes on nutrition, fitness, and the science of sugar.

Well-fed women: a podcast covering intuitive eating, cravings, and health goals.

The keto diet podcast: great for exploring sugar-free recipes and lifestyle strategies.

Feel better, live more with dr. Rangan chatterjee: inspiring conversations about managing cravings and building healthy habits.

The mindbodygreen podcast: expert interviews on mental health, nutrition, and sugar detox tips.

---

4. Templates for habit trackers, food journals, and meal planning

Organizing your progress is a game-changer when it comes to staying accountable and building sustainable habits. Use these templates to track your journey and plan ahead.

Habit tracker

Daily habits:

Water intake (8 glasses per day)
30 minutes of movement (walking, yoga, etc.)
Sugar-free meals and snacks
Sleep (7-9 hours)
Stress management (meditation, journaling)
Weekly reflection:
Wins of the week
Challenges encountered
New habits to focus on next week
Use a physical bullet journal or digital tracking apps like habitbull to log your efforts.
Food journal
Daily log:
Breakfast, lunch, dinner, snacks
Time of meals
How you felt after eating (energy, mood, cravings)
Mood & cravings tracker: note patterns—do certain foods trigger cravings?
Progress review: at the end of each week, reflect on what worked well and areas for improvement.
Keeping a food journal helps you become more mindful of what you're eating and how it affects you, reinforcing healthy choices.
Meal planning template
Weekly planner:
Monday: breakfast – smoothie bowl | lunch – quinoa salad | dinner – baked salmon with roasted vegetables
Tuesday: breakfast – overnight oats | lunch – chicken wrap | dinner – stir-fried tofu with brown rice

Plan out snacks: nuts, boiled eggs, fruit, hummus with carrots.
Shopping list section: fill this in as you plan meals to avoid impulse buys at the store.
Prep day checklist: list the meals and snacks you'll prep in advance (e.g., overnight oats, grilled chicken, chopped veggies).

---

5. Checklist for staying sugar-free long-term

Use this checklist as a roadmap to stay committed to your sugar-free lifestyle and navigate challenges with ease.

Daily habits:
Drink at least 8 glasses of water.
Eat balanced meals with protein, healthy fats, and fiber to stabilize blood sugar.
Avoid processed foods—stick to whole, natural ingredients.
Practice mindful eating: eat slowly and savor your food.
Track cravings and emotional triggers in a food or mood journal.
Weekly habits:
Meal prep healthy snacks and meals to prevent temptation.
Review food labels to spot hidden sugars.
Engage in physical activity at least 4–5 times a

week.
Check in with your goals—are your habits sustainable? Adjust as needed.
Monthly habits:
Reflect on your wins and challenges from the past month.
Experiment with new recipes to keep meals exciting.
Reassess your sugar substitutes—are they helping or triggering cravings?
Celebrate milestones with non-food rewards.
Emergency strategies:
If cravings hit hard, distract yourself: go for a walk, drink herbal tea, or call a friend.
Keep sugar-free snacks on hand—like almonds, yogurt, or an apple—to avoid impulse eating.
If you relapse, don't beat yourself up. Refocus on your next meal or habit and keep moving forward.

---

6. Final thoughts: equipping yourself for success

The resources, tools, and strategies outlined in this bonus section are designed to make your sugar detox and long-term commitment feel manageable and enjoyable. Staying sugar-free isn't about deprivation—it's about empowerment, balance, and making food choices that nourish your body and mind.
When you're well-prepared with healthy foods, apps for accountability, and templates to track your progress, you'll be better equipped to handle cravings and avoid setbacks. Stick with your new habits, celebrate small victories, and use these resources as your go-to guide whenever challenges arise.
Your sugar-free journey isn't just a phase—it's the foundation for a healthier, more vibrant future. And with the right tools in hand, you're ready to thrive!

ABOUT THE AUTHOR

Evelyn started her professional life with a degree from Stanford University. She has taught in several universities and teaching hospitals. She now has her own practice where she takes care of people with many varied emotional issues. She lives alone following the death of her husband, with two large dogs (Rufus and Remus) in a rural community. If she ever has spare time she paints watercolors, and plans to exhibit one day.

Breaking Free from Sugar: A Complete Guide to Reducing Sugar for a Healthier Life

Cut Sugar, Curb Cravings, and Rediscover Your Natural Energy
Sugar Detox

ISBN: 9798345275061

Cover design by Lynnie Ceniza
Interior design and formatting by Lynnie Ceniza
Published by Arthur Crandon Publishing
Visit our website: Arthurcrandon.co.uk

DISCLAIMER

The information provided in this book is for general informational purposes only. It does not constitute legal, financial, or professional advice. While every effort has been made to ensure accuracy, the author and publisher assume no responsibility for errors or omissions. Readers should consult with appropriate professionals for specific advice tailored to their individual circumstances.
First Edition: August 2024